Why Asian women
have symptom-free

MENOPAUSE

And how to be like them!

Dr. Rafael Bolio, MD

First edition

DISCLAIMER

Rafael Bolio is a medical doctor duly registered in his native country Mexico. This book does not dispense medical diagnosis or advice or prescribe the use of any technique as a form of treatment for physical, emotional, or medical problems without the advice of a physician, either directly or indirectly. The intent is only to offer information of a general nature to help you in your quest for emotional, physical, and spiritual well-being. If you use any information in this book for yourself, the author assumes no responsibility for your actions.

ISBN:

DEDICATION

This book is dedicated to those women who followed faithfully my nutritional advice and shared their responses to the plan, including how they went through menopause symptom-free.

Table of Contents

ACKNOWLEDGMENTS

I want to thank Dr. Rafael Camacho Solis, Sub Secretary of State, and Dr. Octaviano Dominguez, Director of Promotion of Health, for entrusting me with creating a nutritional program to help people obtain better health through their personal food choices and control or reduce their blood glucose, cholesterol, triglycerides, blood pressure, volume, and weight. It was thanks to their support and guidance that we were able to create and apply this program successfully at the IMSS (Mexican Institute for Social Security), which provides medical attention to over 40 million people. I also want to thank Dr. Eduardo Garcia Hassey, a doctorate in Psychology, who worked on the emotional component of our project. This program would not have been successful without his expertise and participation.

INTRODUCTION

I smiled when, years ago, I first read that Asian women do not even have a word for menopause.

And why is it that they do they do not even have a word for menopause? Because they go through this phase of life symptom-free.

This was a time when I had to decide what to recommend to over 40 million people in my native country, Mexico.

And I had a human laboratory with over 10,000 personnel in three adjacent office buildings.

These were the main offices of the IMSS (Mexican Institute for Social Security), and the nation's top executives worked there and created action plans for the rest of the country.

I was their doctor, but not only that, I was responsible for keeping them healthy through a program called "Fomento a la Salud" (I am loosely translating it as Promotion of Health).

Most of the personnel were middle-aged men and women, so I had the fantastic opportunity to try out my nutritional approach and discover what it did to my female perimenopause crowd.

This is what I found:

They reduced or normalized the blood glucose, cholesterol, triglycerides, HD, LDL, and blood pressure.

They lost weight and volume.

They maintained and even recovered soft skin and shiny hair.

They reported more energy.

They recovered firm breasts, even if they had been without a period for years.

Their glutes got firmer.

They looked younger.

Their sex drive increased.

Their dry genitals became lubricated again.

They had NO OR MINIMAL SYMPTOMS of menopause: no flushing, no emotional turmoil, nothing.

It became clear that the right nutritional plan helps women endure this period efficiently.

And this is why I smiled when I read that Asian women do not even have a name for menopause.

In this book, I will review what Asian women do, and it would be wise if you consider this information when planning your daily meals.

PART ONE will come with numbers. If numbers make you dizzy, go directly to **PART TWO** of this book and start your meal plan. Even if you need help understanding why the program works, it does not matter if it works for you.

I will first review what Asian women do nutrition-wise compared to American women. Afterward, I will present a simplified program to help you reduce and possibly eliminate menopausal symptoms.

I focused solely on women living in Japan. However, women from other Asian countries share many things we will review.

Why Japanese women? Because Japan has the highest life expectancy in the world. And who knows? By adopting some of their excellent habits, you can also prolong your days here on earth in a happy, healthy way!

You do not need to have been born in Asia or change countries to obtain these benefits. All you have to do is follow the plan outlined in the book.

It will take some time for this program to take effect before you feel fantastic. If you want to "tough it out," you can.

But if you are now suffering from severe menopause symptoms, please go to your doctor and ask them for treatment. When the program takes effect, you can reduce or eliminate these meds or supplements.

How fast can you get results?

This is variable and depends on how well-nourished you are before starting.

Some see results in two or three weeks. In others, it could take two to three months. Finally, there will be some women who will not find benefit, but what do you have to lose from creating a meal plan that has many of the fantastic habits of Asian women?

I will be comparing the following: Life expectancy, Weight and Volume, Diet, and Exercise.

And even if you discover that it extremely difficult to transform yourself into an Asian woman, do not worry because you will find a simplified way of getting the same results with less effort in PART TWO of this book.

For those who love numbers, let us start:

PART ONE

LIFE EXPECTANCY

Japan has the longest life expectancy in the world. Men live an average of 81.5 and women an average of 87.6 years! (1)

America has the worst life expectancy of all developed countries (2).

How far off are we? Men in America live 8.3 years less than men living in Japan. Women living in America live 8.5 years less than women living in Japan.

WEIGHT

The average weight of Japanese middle-aged women is 117 lb. (3)

The average weight of middle-aged American women is 176.4 lb.

Yikes! Japanese women beat American women weight-wise by a long shot! Almost a 60-pound difference!

HEIGHT

The average Japanese middle-aged woman is 0.7 inches shorter than the average American woman. (4)

This height difference does not explain the considerable difference in weight between Japanese and American middle-aged women.

VOLUME

The average waist size for middle-aged Japanese women is 29.5 inches (5)

The average waist size for middle-aged American women is 39.4 inches (6).

Again, Japanese middle-aged women come out much better regarding a trim waistline. Their waistlines are 10 inches smaller than in America!

NUTRITION:

Perhaps the way Japanese people eat is why they have the longest life span in the world and why Japanese women have none or minimal menopause symptoms. Let's review these differences:

ANIMAL PROTEIN

The graphs below report the kilograms of protein that each country eats per person per year (7).

People living in Japan eat more animal protein from the ocean as you can see in the following table:

Country	Poultry	Pork	Fish & Seafood	Bovine	Mutton & Other
Jamaica	53.9	3.1	25.2	3.8	0.7
Jordan	26.1	0.0	5.1	6.8	4.8
Japan	22.3	21.3	46.2	9.6	0.3

Americans eat more poultry and beef than the Japanese, as you can see in the following table.

Country	Poultry	Pork	Fish & Seafood	Bovine	Mutton & Other
Tanzania	1.5	0.3	6.4	7.8	1.6
Ukraine	24.9	16.7	13.8	7.2	0.7
Uganda	1.5	2.9	14.3	3.6	1.0
U.S.	58.7	30.6	22.8	37.9	1.4

The type of animal protein is different, and the total amount is different. In total, the Japanese eat 99.43 kilograms of animal protein per year. Americans eat a total of 151.4 kilograms of animal protein per year. Wow!

Here is a graph where you can see the differences more clearly:

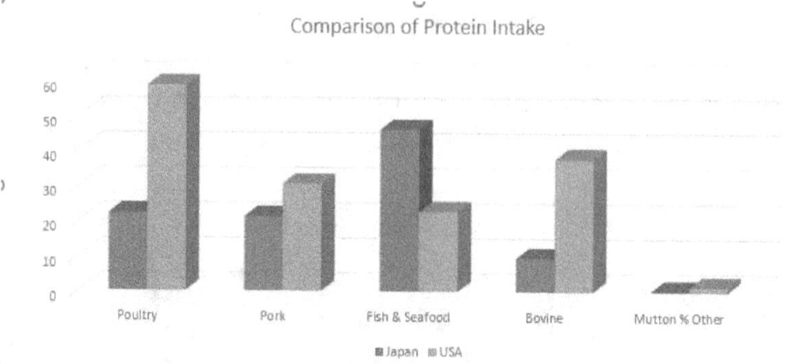

MILK AND MILK PRODUCTS (YOGURT)

Middle-aged Japanese men and women have an average milk and milk products consumption of 3.9 ounces per day on average (8)

Middle-aged American men and women have an average milk consumption of 7.5 ounces daily.

People living in Japan drink very little milk and milk products.

CHEESE:

Japan consumes an average of 6 pounds of cheese per person per year. (9).

According to the US Department of Agriculture Economic Research Service, the average US consumer ate about 40.2 pounds of cheese in 2020.

Wow! Americans eat 6.7 times more cheese!

VEGETABLES

The variety of vegetables that Japanese women eat is extraordinary! I will list the 10 most common vegetables eaten daily, and guess what? They do not even include lettuce, tomatoes, potatoes, or spinach!

On average, they eat 4 to 6 cups of vegetables per day (10)

See if you know or have eaten any of these:

1. Negi: Japanese Bunching Onion

2. Kabocha: Kabocha Pumpkin

3. Daikon: Mooli

4. Shiso: Perilla

5. Naga-imo: Japanese Mountain Yam

6. Renkon: Lotus Root

7. Takenoko: Bamboo Shoots

8. Wasabi

9. Gobo: Burdock Root

10. Satsuma-imo: Sweet Potato

In America, less than 10% of the population eats even the minimum daily recommended vegetable intake of 2 to 3 cups daily. What is the average? 1.2 cups per day, ugh! (11).

Now, out of those measly vegetables that we do eat, this is what people in America choose (12):

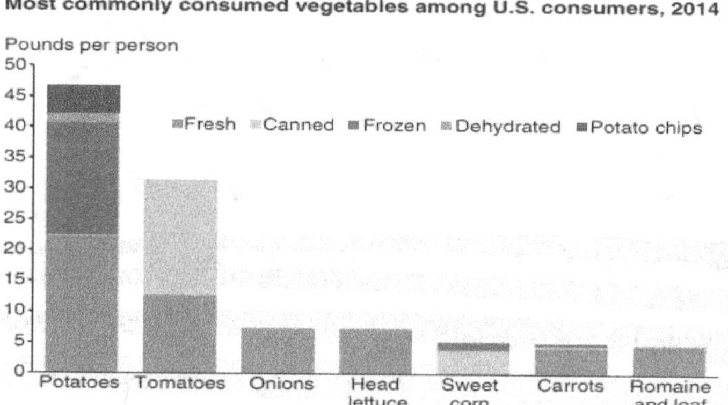

Loss-adjusted food availability data are proxies for consumption.
Source: USDA, Economic Research Service, Loss-Adjusted Food Availability Data.

Potatoes and tomatoes make up for over 75% of our vegetables! We are indeed a country that ignores vegetables altogether. And you still wonder why we are the country that dies the fastest among developed countries?

FRUITS

People living in Japan eat 33.5 kilograms of fruit per person annually, which is very low (13).

Fruit supply per person
kilograms per year per capita

Country or region ⇅	1961	2020	Absolute Change
Jamaica	117.33 kg	134.48 kg	+17.15 kg
Japan	29.12 kg	33.51 kg	+4.39 kg

Americans eat more fruit than in Japan, with an average of 93.75 kilograms per person yearly.

Fruit supply per person
kilograms per year per capita

Country or region	1961	2020	Absolute Change
United Kingdom	54.78 kg	86.40 kg	+31.62 kg
United States	81.13 kg	93.75 kg	+12.62 kg

FERMENTED FOODS

Japan has been called the "Mother of Fermented Foods" (14). It is easy to see why (15):

Natto

Miso

Shoyu

Tsukemono

Umeboshi

Katsuobushi

Kimchi

Yakult

Kefir

Yogurt.

The first six are eaten daily.

America is just finding out that fermented foods exist, and those traditionally created by fermentation, such as yogurt and beer, are pasteurized and do not have the live bacteria to help us obtain better health.

Less than 10% of Americans eat fermented foods with live bacteria on a daily basis, and 90% come from only two sources: kombucha and yogurt (16).

Japan won, and America lost in the competition to use fermented foods in daily meals. Could this tremendous difference be the most critical component for obtaining symptom-free menopause? You will find out for yourself!

SEAWEED

Seaweed is used in 20% of daily dishes in Japan (17)

Americans know about seaweed, but the consumption is so low that I found no scholarly article reporting how much is eaten here in the USA.

RICE

Japanese eat 82.1 kg of rice per year (18).

Americans eat 10.8 kilograms per year.

Interesting! In Japan, people eat almost eight times more rice and weigh much less than Americans, with a plus that they have trimmer waistlines and live longer! I suspect convincing Japanese people to eat less rice to trim their waistline will be extremely difficult.

LEGUMES

Japanese men and women eat an average of 50 grams of legumes daily (19).

Americans eat an average of 20 grams of legumes daily.

We consume tiny amounts of legumes: beans, lentils, chickpeas, peas, soybeans, and fava beans.

I am confident you know these legumes, but statistics show they are not essential to your diet.

TOTAL CARBS

Middle-aged Japanese women eat 59.7% of total carbs daily (20).

Carb intake has plummeted in America from 50.7% to 46.7% in the past 16 years (20).

46.7% is considered a low-carb diet. The low-carb craze is getting worse and worse here in the USA.

Taking into consideration that we have the shortest life span of all developed countries and that Japan eats six times more rice than we do, it is wise to consider that our carb reduction might not be helping us live longer.

SALT:

Middle-aged Japanese people eat an average of 10 grams of salt per day! (21)

Middle-aged American people eat an average of 3.4 grams per day. (22)

Even when people living in Japan can include much more salt and live longer, we must follow what our doctors tell us to do, especially if we have high blood pressure.

FATS

Total fat intake in Japanese middle age women is 26 to 28% of calories per day (23)

Total fat intake in Americans is 35% of calories per day (24)

Americans eat less carbs and more fats, and what is that doing to the country? Nothing good considering menopause symptoms and lifespan that is for sure.

SUGAR

People living in Japan consume an average of 17.23 grams of sugar per person per day (25)

Americans consume an average of 33.17 grams of sugar per person per day

Americans eat or drink twice as many sugars as people living in Japan. And even when Americans eat a double portion of sugars, percentage of total carbs is very low compared to Japan. Americans eat or drink more sugar; Japanese eat more rice.

FASTING

96% of women living in Japan eat 3 meals per day, and 76% have daily snacks. They do not have a fasting routine. (26)

When people living in Japan fast, it is only for religious reasons during Ramadan (27) and very few people living in Japan are Muslims.

10% of people in America follow an intermittent fasting to control their weight. It is the most popular diet trend (28).

Intermittent fasting is becoming the newest diet trend in the USA. Still, people from Japan show us that we do not need to fast to have the longest life span in the world, healthy weight, thin waistline, and symptom-free menopause.

CALORIES

Japanese middle-aged women eat an average of 1,800 to 2,000 calories daily (29).

I did not find a trustworthy online source for calorie intake in middle-aged American women for 2022. The latest report I found comes from the NHANES study from the year 2000 (30), which states that middle-aged women ate about 2000 calories per day.

So, if we consider this previous information, Japanese and American middle-aged women eat the same amount of food in calories, however, with differences in total carbs, fats and type of protein.

EXERCISE

People living in Japan do not like programmed exercise. More than half of the nation does not exercise at all. And the 20% of those who report that they exercise do it either once a week or once a month. All they do is walk, and even then, it is not seen as programmed exercise because it is part of their daily routine (31). They walk an average of 7,000 steps per day (32).

In America, one out of five people report that they exercise regularly (33). Of those who do exercise, half state that they walk. So, only one out of ten Americans walk as the preferred form of exercise on a regular basis.

And even then, as a nation, we walk between 3,000 and 4,000 steps daily, considered sedentary (34). We are an inactive country.

Japan, which has no exercise culture, moves more than people in America, despite so many exercise facilities and commitment to work out.

SUMMARY

Middle-aged women living in Japan eat very differently from American middle-aged women.

This, for me, is the main reason they go symptom-free through menopause.

Why do I state this? Because I observed similar results with middle-aged women when they followed my meal plan.

Let us mention the differences between what middle-aged women do in America and what Japan does as a nation, nutrition and exercise-wise:

Japanese middle-aged women eat as many calories as American women, do not exercise, and yet weigh less, have less abdomen, and have no or minimal symptoms during menopause. Plus, they live longer and healthier.

Women living in Japan do not fast; when they do, it is for religious reasons, not to reduce menopause symptoms.

People in America eat only two vegetables regularly, one is potatoes, and the other tomatoes. Japanese men and women eat an average of over ten vegetables daily.

People living in Japan also eat almost three times more cups of vegetables per day people in America.

They eat at least six fermented foods daily. The only fermented foods that very few from America include are kombucha and yogurt.

They eat more fish than other animal proteins. Americans eat more chicken.

People in Japan eat more carbs, including 2 ½ times more legumes and 7 times more rice than in the USA.

This high grain and legume consumption helps them eat more plant-based protein than women living in America.

People in Japan use seaweed to savor their food. Americans rarely eat seaweed.

They eat less total fat than in America.

They eat half the sugar Americans consume.

The only eating habit that is better in women living in America is salt consumption.

They do not exercise regularly, but they have such an active lifestyle that they walk an average of 7,000 steps daily. Here in the USA, 20% exercise regularly, yet the average steps are 3,00 to 4,000 per day, which amounts to a sedentary lifestyle.

Fortunately, you do not have to do EVERYTHING they do.

The successful program I created for the IMSS shares similar food choices, and even when I was not focusing on menopause, it became a fantastic tool to avoid or reduce symptoms.

What were my patients instructed to eat that is similar to what women in Japan eat?

The program consisted of 50 to 60% carbs, similar to what people eat in Japan. Fats were 28 to 32%, similar to what people eat in Japan. Protein was 15% which was identical for both countries.

People were instructed to continue eating corn, corn-based foods, and beans. This helped them eat more plant-based protein than animal-based protein.

People in Japan obtain their plant-based protein from rice.

In Mexico we have corn, so I used corn as the basis for grains instead of rice. They could eat rice if they wanted, but their preference was corn and corn-based foods.

I learned from women in Mexico that corn is as useful as rice to lessen menopause symptoms.

Women in Japan eat 60 grams of legumes per day which is about ½ cup. People in Mexico usually eat more legumes, and sometimes they eat up to three cups per day. My recommendation was to eat legumes at least twice a day.

They were instructed to eat at least 4 cups of a variety of veggies per day, similar to what people eat in Japan.

PART TWO of this book gives you a doable program based on the diet plan that helped thousands of women go symptom free through menopause and that I hope you will adopt for the rest of your life

The best part is that you do not have to eat exactly what middle-aged women in Japan eat.

You do have to make some important changes to your daily plate, but if you follow the plan, you should come out with choices that are easy and enjoyable.

If we focus on what is most important, we should create a wonderful meal plan that makes us as healthy as people living in Japan.

So let us put on our willpower hat, grab our veggies and fermented foods, and let us move on to a better nutritional lifestyle.

Let us advance to PART TWO:

PART TWO

THE FOUR PHASES

The program is divided into four phases. They are:

PHASE ONE:

The habit changing phase.

PHASE TWO:

The fast weight-loss phase.

PASE THREE

The restoration phase.

PHASE FOUR

The variety phase.

Let us go through a quick summary of each one:

PHASE ONE

Why do people in America eat such few vegetables? Because they do not enjoy them.

Phase one has been created to help you add new foods and make them so enjoyable that you never stop eating them.

You should fall in love with your veggies and fermented foods. If you do not, sooner or later, you will abandon the best part of the plan.

PHASE ONE was created to change not only the variety and frequency of vegetables and fermented foods but also your taste buds so that you enjoy them so much that you cannot live without them.

Each veggie has a special taste that we can focus on to easily find our love for it.

But fermented foods are something else. You need to repeat and repeat them until you get to the point where you accept their bitter flavor. It is also tough to get used to their aroma.

You will have to exert you resolve and continue with fermented foods until you finally accept them.

You can and need to get to the point where you truly enjoy these two food groups.

PHASE TWO

This phase answers the following question: can middle aged women lose their excess fat without drooping all over and looking older than when they started?

It can and should be done and precisely this is what phase two does. It helps you walk the thin line between fast weight loss and the loss of things you do not want to lose.

I want you to keep your figure and even rejuvenate it. It can be done but you have to follow the rules for stage two like your beautiful body depended on it. Because it does.

Another benefit from balanced diets is that they help you lose more waistline than other parts of your body.

You can repeat phase two as many times as you want, but sooner or later you should change this repetitive diet.

You usually lose a lot of weight from PHASE ONE, and PHASE TWO should help you consolidate the process.

PHASE THREE

This phase answers the following question: can you recover the youthful parts of your body that you lost?

Since a balanced nutrition can help you recover firm breasts and tight glutes, it would be useful for you to learn this strategy.

If you do not want to look younger, you do not have to apply PHASE THREE, but I recommend that you follow it just to learn to do it right. This way if you lost something you should not from your body, you can come back to this phase to recover things.

A weight loss program cannot be only about losing weight. It is about losing it the right way.

When you get to this phase, you will understand clearly what this fuss is all about.

PHASE FOUR

Phase four answers the following question: can a weight loss program be so much fun that I never want to leave it?

It can, and that is what phase four is about. Eating balanced meals can not only be healthy, it can be fun!

Each phase has its own special characteristics. You can repeat any of these phases and even go back and forth from one to another.

I do want to advance that PHASE THREE and FOUR will most probably make you lose weight and volume more slowly.

Do you want to advance to the next phase and lose weight and volume more slowly but recover a youthful body?

Or do you want to go back to a phase where you lost a lot of weight and volume?

I leave this decision up to you.

PHASE ONE

Habit changing phase

SMOOTHIE NUMBER ONE (1200 balanced calories)

1 measuring scoop of veggie or whey protein powder (15 grams)

¼ cup walnuts (30 grams)

½ measuring cup of raw oats (40 grams)

1 heaping tablespoon of cocoa powder (10 grams)

2 tablespoons of hulled hemp seeds (20 grams)

1 tablespoon of ground flax seeds, chia seeds, or psyllium plantago (10 grams)

6 ounces of low-fat kefir, any fruit flavor (170 grams)

1 cup of fresh or frozen blueberries (100 grams)

½ cup of fresh or frozen cherries (80 grams)

1 cup of fresh or frozen strawberries (200 grams)

1 medium banana (120 grams)

Add water, divide into 8 equal cups, and drink one cup every 2 to 3 hours

DAY ONE: Prepare your smoothie and divide it into 8 identical cups; drink one cup every 2 to 3 hours. If you want to lose weight and volume faster, divide the smoothie into 12 equal cups and drink one cup every hour. Drink at least 8 extra cups of water during the day. You can use plain water, coffee, or any type of tea all day long.

If you absolutely despise a specific fruit from the smoothie, change it for a fruit you love. Still, your menopause symptoms might disappear a little slower.

In case you feel famished after drinking your smoothie, add any of the vegetables indicated for DAY TWO.

DAY TWO: Add as many different vegetables as you can from the following list: arugula, beets, broccoli, carrots, any onion, celery, cucumbers, organic spinach, green leaves including all kinds of lettuce, any mushrooms, any potatoes, zucchini. Eat them cooked or raw. Season with garlic, salt, pepper, and any other condiment. Add miso paste and/or seaweed leaves if you decide to make a soup.

Eat them every two to four hours and chew them completely.

If you are not used to eating veggies, start with small amounts. Variety is more important than volume this week. People who do not eat veggies might get stomach issues when adding them. If this happens to you, consider adding broad-spectrum digestive enzymes to reduce symptoms. Try one or two capsules four times a day, and if issues persist, check with your doctor to ensure it is not more serious than just an adjustment to veggies.

Continue with your smoothie from day one.

DAY THREE: Add the following fruits: berries, mangoes, organic apples, pears, and stone fruits (peaches, nectarines, plums, apricots, dates, and cherries). If you are not used to eating fruits, moderate them like your veggies to reduce digestive issues. If necessary, add digestive enzymes.

Continue with your smoothie and veggies from day two.

DAY FOUR: Add more fermented foods. You are already drinking kefir and using prebiotics (fiber), which feed your good bacteria. Add raw sauerkraut, raw kimchi, kombucha, yogurt with live active cultures, Greek yogurt, kefir, tempeh, natto, kvass, beer (Belgian or IPA) and any other fermented vegetable like fermented pickles. Consider olives and capers. Eat any of these at least three times per day, except for kvass and beer that contain alcoholic.

Continue with the smoothie, veggies, and fruits.

DAY FIVE: Add fish or shellfish to any meal. Eat at most 12 cooked ounces of salmon and tuna per week. This day, you will also include extra virgin olive oil for salads, extra light olive oil for cooking, avocado, walnuts, and coconut oil. You can cook veggies and fish with extra light olive oil to make things more flavorful.

Continue with the smoothie, vegetables, fruits, and fermented foods.

DAY SIX: Add at least ½ cup of peas. They are legumes to rotate for lentils, chickpeas, and beans later on. If you do decide to add beans on this day, consider that you are already eating a lot of fiber, and you do not want to get an upset stomach. Keep some broad-spectrum digestive enzymes handy to solve any "gassy" issues with peas.

Continue with the smoothie, vegetables, fruits, fermented foods, fish and shellfish.

DAY SEVEN: Add at least ½ cup of cooked rice to meals. You can even add some fermented natto, which is how Japanese women spice up their rice. Add minimal natto because getting used to the taste takes time!

Continue with the smoothie, vegetables, fruits, fermented foods, fish, and peas.

INSTRUCTIONS FOR PHASE ONE:

Prep your smoothie like this: include all dry products in one plastic bag and fruits in another. Freeze your fruits bag. Do this for all seven smoothies of the week. This reduces time preparation to less than 5 minutes per day. Add the bag with dry ingredients, the bag with frozen fruits, kefir, and blend!

Add enough water to make a 32-ounce super smoothie. Remember that you are going to divide it into 8 equal cups. Depending on how thick you want your smoothie, you can add more or less water.

Dividing the smoothie into twelve equal cups and drinking one cup every hour could make you lose weight and volume faster.

Drink lots of extra water, which can help you feel less hungry. The smoothie has 1,200 calories and could help you feel satiated for a day or two. But just in case, add coffee, any tea, and as much water as possible (alkaline, structured, spring, seltzer, hot, cold, etc.).

Now, if on day one you are starving despite drinking the smoothies and lots of extra water, add any of the vegetables recommended for DAY TWO. Even when you add these veggies, you are still going on a plan that helps you eliminate toxins.

Remember that if veggies cause gut issues, you can add digestive enzymes.

If you are still famished after adding veggies, increase the fruits outlined for DAY THREE. The smoothie plus veggies and fruits can give you a lot of calories. If, on day one, you end up eating all that was programmed for days two and three, advance to DAY FOUR.

On **DAY TWO**, you will start biting on lots of different veggies, and previous fast should help you enjoy what you eat, which are veggies, and hopefully, adding lots of different ones will also be fun.

The slight hunger created by day two should help you with this. And you know how hunger makes things taste better!

Chew on your veggies, focus on their flavor and enjoy!

Focus on their taste and have a good conversation with yourself saying that this is going to become a lifelong habit.

There are three easy ways to increase vegetable variety:

NUMBER ONE: create a delicious vegetable soup. Include as many veggies as possible. Cook them with either beef or chicken or vegetable broth and add any condiment to make it taste even better. A fantastic effect of cooked veggies is that the volume of leafy vegies is reduced. I have calculated that a cup of cooked vegetable soup contains as much as five cups of raw veggies.

NUMBER TWO: blend your veggies. Start your blended veggie trip with the current list, and afterwards be creative and add whatever new veggie you want.

Perhaps day two is not the best for blending veggies, but on day three, when you add fruits, you can blend them together and some combinations can be absolutely delicious.

Here is one fantastic blend of veggies with fruit:

½ cup of raw watercress

½ cup of raw spinach

¼ cup of raw cilantro

¼ cup of raw parsley

1 cup of berries, fresh or frozen

Add water

NUMBER THREE: put your veggies through a juicer. This is probably the most complicated one because you need to buy a juicer to make it happen.

This is the option that concentrates veggies the most; you can concentrate up to ten cups of veggies into a single cup of juice.

The taste of the extract, just like the blended veggies is harsh on the palate, but fruit juices can make things way easier on your palate.

Of the three options, the easiest to turn into a habit is soup and the hardest is juicing.

On **DAY THREE** you will be adding fruits! People in America do not seem to have too much of a problem with eating fruits. This is actually a group that is higher in American than Japanese women. You should have no problem including them in your plan.

A quick word about keto dieters: they seem to satanize fruits as one of the greatest nutritional evils that ever existed. If you are a keto fan, adding fruits could be difficult on the mind, not on the body. Try adding one and weight yourself the next day. If there is no weight gain, you can conclude that at least one a day is okay.

Ideally you should avoid fruit juices, but you can cook your apples, include frozen or dried fruits, and blend your fruits with your vegetables.

On **DAY FOUR**, you will add a food group that I believe, together with including a high variety of vegetables, makes women in Japan the healthiest in the world and helps them go through menopause symptom-free.

Fermented foods are what we call "learned taste." Two examples of learned taste are beer and tobacco. No one can say the first time they try beer that it tastes delicious, and the same goes for tobacco. But once we associate this bitter flavor with a sensation of well-being, we "enjoy" this bitter taste.

The same goes for fermented foods. They do not taste good, but since our good bacteria love being pampered, they send good sensations after you have ingested them. If we repeat fermented foods, we end up loving them. Believe me, it happens!

Start with small quantities, a bite for every meal, and slowly increase them. Eating at least ½ ounce of kimchi can give you all the benefits (35). Just imagine multiplying benefits three times when you eat ½ ounce every meal.

Kimchi is just one option, you also have sauerkraut, kombucha, kefir, Greek yogurt, plain yogurt with live active cultures, tempeh, natto, olives, capers, kvass, Belgian beer (just a little), and fermented pickles.

Preserves made with vinegar do not have probiotics; preserves made with salt do.

On **DAY FIVE**, you will add fish and shellfish. Many of my clients do not like fish and shellfish. This is because they have yet to get used to the flavor. Even if you detest fish and shellfish, eat them; with time, you will learn to love them.

When enticing yourself to eat fish or shellfish, take into consideration that menopause symptoms can be very uncomfortable and last longer than whatever time it takes to learn to enjoy something that you do not like yet.

There is no such thing as bad-tasting vegetables or bad-tasting fish, but there is such a thing as a bad cook. Check for online recipes; vegetables and fish can become extraordinarily delicious platters.

DAY SIX has to do with legumes, another food that some people need to find a way to like. Take into account that legumes and rice are the foods that make people in Japan eat more plant-based protein than Americans, and that can also be part of the reason why they live longer than people in America.

Start with peas and graduate to other legumes. Chickpeas are relatively easy to digest, and so are lentils. Remember to use condiments to make them tastier.

Beans are another story.

To digest them better, leave them covered in water all night long and throw away water the next morning before cooking them. Using a pressure cooker can make it easier for your digestion. Blend or mash your beans; this also helps you have fewer issues.

If nothing seems to work, take one or two capsules of broad-spectrum digestive enzymes before eating them. After one or two weeks, your body should be creating enzymes needed to digest them.

DAY SEVEN adds rice to your plan. Use white, brown, or wild rice. Cook it without using oils, just like in Japan.

How is it that people in Japan eat so much rice? Because they eat rice even at breakfast. You can cook your rice to the point that you create a porridge and add honey to make it taste sweet.

My patients ate lots of corn and corn-based meals like tortillas and other traditional corn-based foods, and they went through menopause symptom free.

I cannot swear that wheat products will also do the job, but you can try them out together with other options like barley, quinoa, amaranth, oats, buckwheat, and teff. Rotating grains is an excellent habit.

EXTRA TIPS

Can you fast for more than one day using only the smoothie from day one?

Can you repeat the whole plan from day one to seven for another week?

Can you stay on day seven for more than one day?

Yes, to all!

If you do repeat any part of this plan, you could transform your face, body, health, and perspective on nutrition in just a few weeks.

But before you decide that you want to make a total transformation in as little time as possible, read the information from PHASE TWO AND THREE:

You should not lose muscle or structural fat.

One week of PHASE ONE has never given me issues concerning loss of muscle or structural fat, but repeating the plan for more than two weeks could cause issues.

Being healthier is not only about losing weight and volume.

If this were so, people with anorexia and bulimia would be the healthiest in the word, and they are not. They are people with severe undernutrition / malnutrition.

Gaining weight and losing it can alter your menstrual cycle and your menopause symptoms (36).

And it gets worse. Women on menopause who go on yo-yo dieting increase their risk of dying from hear attacks (37).

To be the fastest does not always translate to being the best. It is very important that you obtain a clear and continuous loss of weight and volume without ups and downs.

Also take into account that repeating PHASE ONE takes work.

To increase your possibility of success, team up with friends or family and support each other by creating yummy dishes and cheering each other on.

But if these seven days were more than enough for you, let's advance to PHASE TWO:

PHASE TWO

Fast weight loss phase

1,332 TOTAL BALANCED CALORIES

SMOOTHIE TWO (500 balanced calories)

1 measuring scoop of veggie or whey protein powder (20 grams)

16 whole walnuts (20 grams)

1 heaping tablespoon of cocoa powder (10 grams)

1 cup of fresh or frozen blueberries (100 grams)

½ cup of fresh or frozen cherries (80 grams)

1 medium banana (120 grams)

Add water, divide into 4 equal cups, and drink one cup early morning, the second in mid-morning, the third in mid-noon, and the fourth with dinner or after dinner.

BREAKFAST: Fermented food

½ cup of raw oats cooked in water

One tablespoon of honey

Eight walnut halves (10 grams)

LUNCH: Fermented food

At least 2 oz of cooked fish, chicken breast,

low-fat cheese, or 2 eggs

½ medium avocado (80g of pulp) or 2 teaspoons

of extra virgin olive oil

At least 2 cups of vegetables, cooked or raw

Plain water

DINNER: Fermented food

One cup of cooked rice, pasta, or quinoa

½ cup of peas, chickpeas, lentils or beans

¼ medium avocado (40g of pulp) or 1 teaspoon

of extra virgin olive oil

At least 2 cups of any vegetables, cooked or raw

Plain water

Continue with fermented foods in your three main meals: kefir, sauerkraut, kimchi, or pickled veggies.

Always include as many different vegetables as you can. Eat at least 4 cups of veggies per day. Consider adding new vegetables: artichoke hearts, asparagus, Brussels sprouts, watercress, eggplant, bok choi, and any other you want.

Try a different legume each day, and if any of them cause even minor stomach issues, leave them pending for the following weeks.

Consider including a miso soup with seaweed leaves at least three times per week.

Try to use fish and shellfish for three days, chicken for two days, cheese for one day, and beef, pork, two eggs, or turkey one day of the week.

Hopefully this program is easier to follow, and if you feel comfortable, repeat it as many weeks as you want.

INSTRUCTIONS FOR WEEK TWO

WEEK TWO has 1,303 total calories, with 500 calories coming from the new **smoothie two**. It now includes breakfast, lunch, and dinner.

Why is the new smoothie programmed to be taken between meals?

People who eat small snacks between meals can follow low-calorie programs much longer without cheating. Hopefully, these smoothies will do the magic.

Also, SMOOTHIE TWO, just like SMOOTHIE ONE can help you reduce menopause symptoms quickly.

Drink the first cup of this divided smoothie as soon as you wake up, the second one between breakfast and lunch, the third between lunch and dinner, and the last one after dinner.

If still hungry, add more veggies, fruits, probiotics, and fish. Veggies increase your tolerance to strict diets quite well.

Let's talk about **BREAKFAST:**

Measure your oats before cooking. Once you have cooked them with water, you should obtain delicious bowl of oats!

Adding honey and walnuts makes it taste better, and we must include them to balance the 24-hour program.

You can change oats for buckwheat to makes another delicious breakfast. You must also add honey and walnuts.

Add fermented food, and if you choose kefir, Greek

yogurt, or plain yogurt with live active cultures, mix them with your oatmeal or buckwheat.

LUNCH is as simple as it gets. Just protein and veggies.

Protein is not limited; eat as much as you want, but do not eat less than 2 ounces. Try to eat fish or shellfish three days a week, chicken 2 days a week, cheese one day of the week, and on the seventh day, choose beef, pork, or eggs.

Cook your protein any way you want. This plan includes a total of ¾ avocado or 3 teaspoons of extra virgin olive oil. Although you can use oil to cook your protein, you get better results when included in salads or by themselves.

Some veggies generate a faster loss of waistline than others. Lettuce with onions, mushrooms, radishes, and watercress can make your waistline look really great!

Add artichoke hearts, Jerusalem artichoke, asparagus, and any other vegetable that you can to turn into a daily routine. Just be careful with digestive issues from veggies. Prefer variety over quantities.

You now have olive oil and avocado for salads. Avocado is fantastic: just by itself, it can make you lose up to an inch off your waist in three to four weeks. The same goes for mushrooms.

If you need to lubricate your private parts, switch avocado and olive oil for 24 extra walnut halves, preferably raw. If your private parts are really causing issues, add as many walnuts as you can. You can also use almonds. You will lose weight more slowly, but in return, you will get your sexual life back.

Include fermented foods: choose between sauerkraut, kimchi, miso, fermented veggies, kombucha, and kefir for breakfast, lunch and dinner.

You can change your lunch to dinner and dinner to lunch. The order is less important than the fact that you do eat them all.

DINNER: dinner includes foods that are a good source of vegetable protein. It is not a fantastic meal, but you do want 1,300 calories, the sweet spot to lose the most weight and volume in the shortest time possible. Anything under 1,200 calories makes you lose more weight but less volume; anything over 1,300 calories makes you lose more volume but less weight.

You can add animal protein to your dinner. Try repeating the same protein from lunch for an easier digestion.

People in Asia eat lots of rice, but you can use pasta instead as long as there is no wheat intolerance. Also include quinoa and corn. Rotating grains and cereals reduce the possibility of getting gut inflammation.

Be careful with this plan (and any other plan with less than 1,500 calories) because it could make you lose muscle and structural fat.

When this happens, you will almost always recover what you lost and gain even more (the dreaded yo-yo).

Why?

1,300 calories are meager; if a woman burns more than 2,100 calories daily, she might start losing things she should not.

How do you know if you are losing muscle?

Buy a measuring tape for sewist: measure your calf at the widest point. Do this every day. **Measure it in centimeters.** Also, measure your waist in centimeters at your belly button.

It would be best to lose little or no circumference in the calf because it could mean that you are losing muscle.

I have observed that when you lose ½ cm of calf after losing three to four pounds, you continue to lose excess fat and generate stable weight loss.

But suppose someone loses ½ cm and has only lost one pound. In this case, loss of weight and volume almost always stops.

Most of my clients do not even lose ½ cm during their first month of treatment, which is fantastic!

Keep an eye on your glutes. Check your glutes every morning in the mirror. Make sure that they stay where they should. If they start drooping, it is time to increase calories.

Also, squeeze your arms, glutes, and thighs. They should have a firm tone. If they start to lose tone, it is time to increase calories.

If you do things right, you will begin to see the body of a younger woman in the mirror.

What about structural fat?

The easiest way to identify if you are losing structural fat is by observing your breasts and nipples in a mirror.

Stand straight with your shoulder blades pulled back and turn sideways to observe your breasts. If you have not lost structural fat, your nipples should point forward. If your nipples start going down or sideways, you are probably losing structural fat. If this happens, you will stop losing weight and volume, and it will be tough to maintain whatever you lost. It is time to increase calories.

The following image shows what should not happen with your breasts. The one on the left is normal, but the ones to the right are progressively losing structural fat:

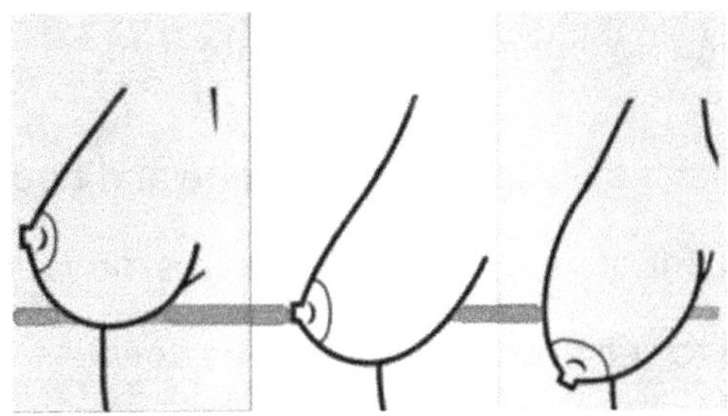

What if you already lost structural fat (sagging breasts) and muscle (flabby glutes) even before starting the plan?

PHASE THREE has the calories that could help you recover youthful breasts and tight glutes.

PHASE THREE will increase to either 1,500 or 1,700 calories.

But do not be afraid of calories. Women living in Japan weigh less and have ten inches less waistline while eating around 2,000 calories per day.

Perhaps you will need to advance to **PHASE THREE** even if you have been on **PHASE TWO** for a few days, which is okay.

Tracking what happens with your program and your body is instrumental. Register weight, number of different veggies you eat per day, number of cups, how many fermented foods you ate, how many times you ate legumes, and how many times you ate fish.

Weigh yourself daily during **phases one and two**. You will likely lose a lot of weight in these phases, and it is motivating to see how your scale goes down.

APPENDIX ONE includes a table where you can write your progress.

Okay, so let's find out what **PHASE THREE** is all about:

PHASE THREE

Recovery phase

1,500 calories without pastry, 1,700 calories with pastry

Early morning: •4 to 6 ounces of flavored kefir (strawberries, blueberries, mango, etc.)

Breakfast: •Fermented food with:
• ½ cup oats or buckwheat (measure raw)
•1 cup 2% fat milk
•8 almonds or 4 whole walnuts
•½ tablespoon of honey
-or-
•½ to 1 medium bagel
 •½ to 1 ounce of regular cream cheese
-or-
•2 eggs in any style (no added oil)
•2 slices of wheat bread or sourdough or corn tortilla
•A small apple, pear, mango, or any other fruit

Morning snack: Any fruit

Lunch: •Fermented food with:
•2 slices of bread, baguette, or sourdough
•2 ounces of low-fat cheese, or low-fat ham, or tuna canned in water, or chicken breast
 •¼ medium avocado or 1 teaspoon of regular mayonnaise or butter
•Vegetables, salt, pepper, and mustard ad-lib
•1 cup of fruit juice or one large fruit

Snack:	•2 ounces of cake or pastry (Twinky Wonder, chocolate cake, apple pie, coffee cake, small doughnuts, cheesecake, etc.).

Dinner: Fermented food with:
•Vegetable soup or broth with vegetables
•½ cup of cooked rice or pasta or quinoa or corn
•½ cup of legumes: beans, chickpeas, or lentils
•At least 2 cups of cooked or raw vegetables
•½ medium avocado or 2 teaspoons of olive oil, or 2 tablespoons of salad dressing
•1 slice of bread, baguette, or sourdough or corn tortilla
•2 ounces of animal protein
•Plain water, coffee or tea

Always, always, always use as many vegetables as your imagination can include in all your meals.

Always, always, always use fermented foods, even in small quantities, in all your meals.

Always, always, always rotate your legumes. Do not eat only peas, lentils, or beans.

Always, always, always rotate your grains like rice, pasta, quinoa, and any other grain.

Use miso paste or seaweed to flavor your meals at least three times per week.

Always, always, always rotate your proteins, trying to eat fish and shellfish three days per week.

INSTRUCTIONS FOR PHASE THREE

YES!

You finished phases one and two.

You have been carefully watching and measuring your body so there is no loss of muscle or structural fat. Now you want to advance to a new program.

PHASE THREE is different in three ways: first, it comes without an MRP or smoothie so that your calories only come from regular foods.

Why take off the smoothie?

This is a long-term project that I hope will become a way of life.

Smoothies are a fantastic to balance calories and body changes can be spectacular, but you also have to learn to live without them. They cannot become a lifestyle.

What is going to be your backup if you do not want smoothies or do not have ingredients to prepare them?

This is precisely the focus of the next phases: provide you with a program that can be used as long as you want to.

If for whatever reason you decide that you want to continue with PHASE TWO, that is okay as long as you are careful to avoid the loss of muscle and structural fat.

And even if for some reason you messed up and lost muscle and structural fat in PHASE TWO, you now have PHASE THREE that can help you recover whatever you lost.

The second difference is that you will be able to choose from three different breakfasts.

You have oats with walnuts and honey for breakfast, just like WEEK TWO, but now you cook your oats with 2% fat milk. If you are milk intolerant, you can use almond, coconut, or rice milk.

You can also have a bagel with cream cheese or eggs with veggies, plus bread or tortilla and a fruit.

All three breakfast choices are almost identical in calories. No matter which one you choose, you are eating around 1,500 calories per day.

The third difference is that you now have a sandwich at lunch. Sandwiches are easy to prepare and easier to carry around. It should make this meal simple to do.

Animal protein in dinner is placed at the end of all other foods. This might help you eat less animal protein without feeling deprived. When you eat your animal protein at the end, you usually eat less than if you eat it at the beginning.

We do not want to eat less total protein. What we want to do is eat more vegetable protein, which is what women in Japan do.

You increase calories a little and this should make it easier to follow the diet and, most important, reduce the risk of slowing down your metabolism because you lost muscle and structural fat.

You have to decide between 1,500 calories and avoiding pastry or going up to 1,700 calories with a yummy dessert!

A special note for your mid-noon pastry:

My experience with hundreds of peri-menopausal women is that when they add pastry to a balanced meal plan, their mammary glands become firmer and tighter, so if they were drooping, they go back up again!

If one slice of pastry is not working, add 2 more ounces. Watch your breasts and see if it is creating magic.

This may happen or not, but having something sweet can make your meal plan much more fun.

If you avoid pastry, you will have increased 1,300 to only 1,500 daily calories.

Middle-aged American women eat an average of 2,000 calories per day. Sooner or later, you will get hungrier and that is okay.

You do not want to eat fewer calories than you should and end up with sarcopenia (loss of muscle mass) which is almost always appears by age 60.

Why would you want to create sarcopenia before hitting 60?

Go up to 1,700 calories by including your pastry as soon as possible. You might not lose excess weight as quickly as you would with less calories, which is okay. We want to look great at 40, 50, 60 and onward.

Another way to increase calories without pastry is with this new smoothie:

SMOOTHIE NUMBER THREE

10 grams of veggie or whey protein powder

One medium banana

Eight walnut halves

One teaspoon of brown sugar or honey

Add water and blend all ingredients.

This smoothie will give you 230 balanced calories which is similar to what you get with 2 ounces of pastry.

If you have increased your calories to 1,700 per day and notice that you are still hungry, you can to hike your plan up to 1,900 to 2,000 calories with another smoothie or another slice of cake.

You can also take a peek at PHASE FOUR where you find other ways to increase calories and continue to have a meal plan that is similar to what middle-aged women eat in Japan.

What to do with all the other yummy dishes we love that are not in this program?

Can we add mac-and-cheese, hamburgers, pizzas, tamales, sushi rolls, popcorn, potato chips, lasagna, hummus, etc.?

Yes! Add whatever you want in two free means per week.

Here is an example: You are having breakfast with friends, so what do you order? Eggs Benedict? Yes. Pancakes? Of course! Add butter and maple syrup or honey. It is one of two free meals.

Here is another example: you have this big dinner, and the food is delicious. Eat whatever you want.

You still lose weight and volume as long as you are disciplined with the rest of you plan. Having two free meals does not mean being disastrous the rest of the week. If you stop losing weight, it is because you are not doing the program right.

Before you advance to this option, wait for menopause symptoms to disappear or subside.

Are there other ways to increase calories safely? Yes, and we will present them in PHASE FOUR.

PHASE FOUR
The variety phase.

This phase is going to bring you many options.

When you read this chapter, you will find it overwhelming.

Take a deep breath, calm down, and come back to this chapter after you have allowed at least some part of the information to sink in.

Why is it that this chapter can be overwhelming? How we eat is complex, and trying to make sense of so much variety can be exhausting.

Read this chapter one, two, or three times. Every new time, more things will make sense, and you will find yourself empowered with many wonderful choices.

The following is only a small list of balanced meals, and you do need to follow the instructions at the end of this chapter before using them:

GREEK YOGURT PARFAIT (311 balanced calories)

½ cup of plain, non-fat Greek yogurt

12 walnut halves

1 cup of blueberries

1 tablespoon of honey

KEFIR SMOOTHIE (246 balanced calories)

1 cup of low-fat, unflavored kefir

1 and ½ tablespoons of honey (30 grams)

COTTAGE CHEESE WITH FRUIT (335 balanced calories)

½ cup of low-fat cottage cheese

One medium banana, apple, or pear

12 walnut halves

1 tablespoon of honey

OATMEAL (334 balanced calories)

½ cup oats, raw, cooked in milk

1 cup whole milk

½ tablespoon of honey

OREO COOKIES (262 balanced calories)

3 Oreo cookies

1 cup of 1% fat milk

NUTELLA WITH BREAD AND MILK (210 balanced calories)

1 slice of bread (1 ounce)

Nutella 1 tablespoon (20g)

4 ounces of 2% fat milk

PIZZA, CHEESE WITH FRUIT JUICE (292 balanced calories)

3 oz slice of thick-crust cheese pizza

 4 oz of any fruit juice

BREAD WITH CHEESE AND FRUIT (260 balanced calories)

1 slice (1 oz) of bread (white, whole wheat, French, pita, etc.)

1 slice (1 oz) of any cheese

1 medium fruit like apple, pear, or banana, or 1 cup of grapes or berries

AVOCADO TOAST (212 balanced calories)

1 oven-roasted corn tortilla

¼ cup mashed beans

¼ medium avocado

½ cup any raw vegetables

1 ounce of cheese, chicken breast, or tuna canned in water

PIZZA, PEPPERONI, DEEP DISH (360 calories)

4 ounces of pepperoni pizza

This meal is balanced, so you can have as many slices as you want without stuffing yourself.

BREAD WITH PEANUT BUTTER, JELLY AND MILK (276 balanced calories)

1 slice (1 oz) of bread (white, whole wheat, French, pita, etc.)

1 tablespoon of peanut butter

1 tablespoon of jam or jelly

½ cup of 1% fat milk

MAC AND CHEESE (207 to 414 balanced calories)

½ to 1 cup of mac and cheese.

This meal is balanced, so you can have as much as you want without stuffing yourself.

FRENCH TOAST (204 balanced calories)

1 French toast (prepared as usual)

½ cup of 1% fat milk

1 tablespoon of honey

2 tablespoons of whipped cream

TAMALES (250 balanced calories)

One beef, pork or chicken tamales (each about 2.3 ounces)

¼ cup of cooked beans

4 ounces of any fruit juice

SUSHI ROLLS (240 to 300 calories)

All sushi rolls are balanced as long as they are not fried, so you can have as many rolls as you want without stuffing yourself.

HUMMUS WITH SOURDOUGH 186 balanced calories)

One ounce of hummus

1.3 ounces of sourdough bread

TACOS AL PASTOR (404 balanced calories)

Two tacos al pastor

8 ounces of any fruit juice

POZOLE - made with pork (251 balanced calories)

1 cup

This meal is balanced, so you can have as many cups as you want without stuffing yourself.

PHO SOUP, with beef (311 balanced calories)

1 bowl of pHo soup with beef

4 ounces of fruit juice

1 tsp. olive oil or 8 walnut halves

GREEK SALAD – average (212 balanced calories)

1 bowl of Greek salad

8 ounces of fruit juice

CORN TORTILLA WITH CHEESE (281 balanced calories)

Three medium corn tortilla

Three ounces of low-fat cheese

CHEESE SANDWICH (192 balanced calories)

Two slices of bread – total 2 ounces

Two slices of low-fat cheese – total 2 ounces

SPHAGETTI WITH MEATBALLS – (452 balanced calories)

One plate of spaghetti with meatballs

Four ounces of fruit juice

POTATO SALAD WITH EGG – (418 balanced calories)

One cup of potato salad

¼ cup of lentils, cooked without butter or oil

INSTRUCTIONS FOR PHASE FOUR

This is quite a list.

I am certain that some combinations seem easy, while others seem like the craziest diet you have ever seen!

Believe me, when I started to analyze the nutritional programs that I was instructed to apply to workers of the IMSS, I almost went crazy.

What I thought was balanced had nothing to do with what I analyzed with Nutritional software.

The nutritional value of these foods comes from the Internet, and many of them have been prepared in restaurants, like pepperoni pizza and pozole.

One huge problem with store-bought meals is their sodium content is quite high, sometimes taking up over 60% of what you should include in your day.

If you know how to prepare these dishes, you can make a healthier plate. You get to choose the ingredients.

You can also check the Internet for recipes, but you must get into your kitchen and work!

You can buy some of these options from restaurants, but to be safe, do it occasionally.

Some are really complicated to make at home, like tamales, so I would recommend that you buy them.

Why should we worry about including so much variety?

Do we have to? Of course not.

But then, no two people eat the same way, and even the same person can eat different foods from one day to another.

The calories that you need can also change from one month to another. You could be a woman who begins a job with a heavy physical workload. Such is the case for cleaners, chiropractors, physical therapists, etc.

If you burn more energy, you need more calories than an average American woman. This could make 1,700 calories per day more miserable than a satisfying program.

Your appetite can even change from one day to another.

This is the norm and not the exception. On some days, we want more food; others, we want less.

When a diet has a high content of vegetables, fiber, and fermented foods, these spikes are less pronounced, and hunger is easier to control.

This should make recommendations just fine for most days of the year.

But if your hunger does increase, you can add more food, and if it is balanced, you will continue losing excess fat.

I already added a new smoothie in WEEK THREE to handle hunger pangs.

Smoothies or MRP are great because they can create balanced calories, and most importantly, for weight loss, you continue to lose weight and volume.

Another important fact is that almost any food can be turned into a balanced meal and therefore can help you lose weight and volume.

You may not lose weight and volume as quickly when including hamburgers, but you do get the advantage of creating a varied meal plan that will not bore you.

How can you use these meals?

Check the different options and decide which ones suit your life.

When you have created your personalized list, buy the ingredients to have them at home whenever hunger strikes.

When can you add them?

All three main meals from PHASE THREE are balanced, so you can easily switch any of them for the options on this list.

Can you add them to phase two? Yes! As you increase calories in phase two, you could lose weight and volume slowly, which can help you reduce the risk of losing muscle and structural fat.

Can you add them to phase one if you decide to repeat it?

You can, but leave them for days five to seven.

Many of these balanced meals from this list can be doubled or tripled.

 For example, hummus with sourdough bread has only 186 calories; if you are still hungry, add another ounce of hummus with another slice of sourdough bread.

How many new meals can you add, and how many times can you repeat them?

As many as you need to feel okay. You want to feel satisfied but not stuffed.

It would be best if you also took into account food intolerance.

Some people cannot drink milk because they are lactose intolerant. Still, they can eat cheese and kefir because these products have very little lactose.

Other people are intolerant to lactose and a specific protein from cow's milk. They will not tolerate milk, cheese, or kefir.

These are substitutes for people who are intolerant to cow's milk and cow's cheese:

Use goat milk, goat kefir, goat cheese, or even cheese made from lamb's milk. Lactose and protein intolerance is not cross-reactive to these milks.

You can also try tofu, made from soy, which looks like cheese.

There is another very common food intolerance on the rise, and it is gluten intolerance. These people should reduce or eliminate it from their menu.

For gluten intolerance, you can buy bread that does not contain gluten. Amaranth, oats, flax, potatoes, brown and white rice, buckwheat, soy, corn, tapioca, and teff do not have gluten. Look for breads in your store that are gluten-free. They are similar in nutritional content, so you can easily swap them. You can use these for your grain rotations.

Some of these grains have a different flavor that you can get used to, so you should give any of the new grains more than one taste.

Gluten intolerance is not the same as a gluten allergy. People with gluten allergy cannot even eat gluten-free grains handled in places that process wheat. If you have a gluten allergy, you know that you have to buy products that state clearly on the label "gluten-free."

White sourdough is an interesting wheat bread that causes minimal digestive issues. Try it, and maybe you will find a "new love."

Some people have a terrible problem with their digestion and have an intolerance to multiple foods. This can be caused by a problem called a leaky gut.

WEEK ONE can do wonders for people with leaky gut.

There is a strategy called elemental diet that can help people recover from this.

An elemental diet is a plan where you only drink a product that covers your nutritional needs, and that has a very low probability of causing a histamine reaction in your gut.

SMOOTHIE ONE could give the same results.

But if the smoothie generates inflammation in your gut, it means that you have carbohydrate intolerance.

This could be caused by Candida Albicans or parasites, but your doctor must be the one to diagnose and treat these issues.

A word of caution: if you go crazy with this new list and totally abandon weeks one, two, and three, you MUST continue with these basic rules:

Always, always, always use as many vegetables as you can all day long.

Always, always, always use fermented foods, even in small quantities, in your main meals.

Always, always, always rotate your legumes. Do not eat only peas, lentils, or beans.

Always, always, always rotate your grains like rice, pasta, corn, quinoa, and any other grain.

Use miso paste or seaweed to flavor your meals at least three times per week.

Always, always, always rotate your proteins, trying to eat fish and shellfish three days a week.

FITTING THE PIECES TOGETHER

You have gone through the four phases.

You have obtained good to excellent results.

Your menopause symptoms have been reduced or even eliminated.

Now what? What comes next?

Before we advance to all the wonderful options open to you, you need to answer the following question:

How did I do with each phase?

What is easy? Was it hard?

What did I obtain? What did I learn?

If all were fantastic, you are a very fortunate woman.

But what is most likely is that in one or more phases, things worked less perfectly than you wanted.

This is natural, and it has nothing to do with a lack of resolve or discipline. Life is life, and many things can happen.

When problems hit us, they do not ask if we are ready for them or not. This is just part of being alive.

What should you do when things are really difficult? What if you cannot follow any plan? You might even go through moments where you have absolutely no appetite.

In this case, the best action is to eat whatever you can, balanced or not.

Whatever phase you are going through, try to eat at least a little of anything.

When our body receives some food, even if it is absolutely unhealthy, it will do what It can to keep us going. This way, you lessen the risk of shutting down your metabolism.

When you come out of the problem and start feeling hungry again, if you can, go to PHASE FOUR and choose whatever your body craves.

These options are not for fast weight loss, but they are balanced and can help you recover from whatever you went through.

If you are ready, go to day one of PHASE ONE. This day will help you recover a nourished body and can give you spectacular results. From there, decide what phase you want to do next. It does not matter which one, as long as you do it.

Day one of PHASE ONE is fantastic for other things:

If you have gone through a disastrous weekend or vacation and come back with lots of excess weight and a bloated belly, use day one for one or two days to reset your digestion and lose all your accumulated water weight.

You can also use day one of phase one for the 2 / 5 program: follow a strict plan for two days, and for the rest of the week, eat whatever you want.

 How was PHASE TWO?

Did it help you lose weight and volume? Was it hard or easy to follow? Did you lose muscle or structural fat? How many weeks did you stay in it? Did you cheat a lot?

PHASE ONE AND TWO are the most difficult because you are making a total rehaul of your eating habits. A part of PHASE ONE and all of PHASE TWO is low in calories. It is low in calories, but it can generate fast changes.

Some people do not lose so much weight with PHASE TWO but see great changes in their figure.

Why would someone lose very little weight and a lot of volume? When a person is malnourished and starts eating a balanced diet again, the body starts recovering whatever muscle mass and structural fat had been lost.

I have seen how many women start getting tight glutes even with low-calorie diets. This does not happen to everyone, but if you had tight and beautiful glutes, you might get them back with this phase.

If you are happy with the changes from PHASE TWO, you can repeat it as many times as you want as long as you are not losing muscle or structural fat.

How did you do in PHASE THREE?

Did you increase your calories? Were you so afraid of pastry that you preferred to add Smoothie Three? Did you add another slice of pastry? Did you recover tight glutes and breasts? What is too little or too much food?

What can you do with PHASE THREE?

You could stay on PHASE THREE with 1,500, 1,700, or 2,000 calories as good support for Monday through Friday and eat whatever you want on Saturday and Sunday.

Can you mix and match? Yes!

PHASE ONE and PHASE TWO are strict programs. You could use them as the two days of the 2 / 5 diet plan, where you apply a strict diet on two days and eat freely the rest of the week.

You can also create your fun plan mixing up PHASES TWO OR THREE with options from PHASE FOUR. Enjoy your plan and change things around.

Some food choices should always be present. Let us review them because they can be a useful framework for any diet that you decide to apply:

The following is an outline of the most important actions that you should include in your nutritional plan.

Smoothies One and Two can help reduce menopause symptoms quickly, so I have put them in the first place:

1. Use smoothies One and Two.
2. Include fermented foods in every meal.
3. Consume a wide variety of vegetables.
4. Include at least four cups of vegetables daily.
5. Prefer animal protein from the sea.
6. Make legumes part of your daily routine.
7. Prefer vegetable fats over animal fats.

Once menopause symptoms have subsided or disappeared, you can take Smoothies One or Two off your plan. The order of importance for a sustainable lifestyle should be:

1. Include fermented foods in every meal.
2. Consume a wide variety of vegetables.
3. Include at least four cups of vegetables daily.
4. Prefer animal protein from the sea.
5. Include legumes in at least one of your meals.
6. Prefer vegetable fats over animal fats.

These are sustainable life choices can be included by anyone, no matter their sex or age.

FINAL WORDS

There is magic in food, and we have a clear example from Japan, with the longest lifespan in the world, that has women who go through menopause with minimal or no symptoms.

You can participate in this magic, and it is not that difficult. All you must do is follow the plan.

But then again, it is not a walk in the park.

You do need to retrain your taste buds to absolutely love foods that are not on your daily plate.

And it is okay because, with a little discipline and repetition, you can do it.

Focus on what you must do, enjoy the process, and live happy and symptom-free!

APPENDIX

Day	WEIGHT	CALF	WAIST	# OF VEGGIES	CUPS OF VEGGIES	FERMENTED FOODS	LEGUMES YES/NO	FISH/ SHELLFISH
1				smoothie	smoothie	smoothie	smoothie	smoothie
2								
4								
5								
6								
7								
8								
9								
10								
11								
12								
13								
14								
15								
16								
17								
18								
19								
20								
21								
22								
23								
24								
25								
26								
27								
28								

REFERENCES

1. *How does U.S. life expectancy compare to other countries? - Peterson-KFF Health System Tracker.* (2022, December 6). Peterson-KFF Health System Tracker. https://www.healthsystemtracker.org/chart-collection/u-s-life-expectancy-

2. *The pandemic's effect on the widening gap in mortality rate between the U.S. and peer countries - Peterson-KFF Health System Tracker.* (2020, October 22). Peterson-KFF Health System Tracker. https://www.healthsystemtracker.org/brief/the-pandemics-effect-on-the-widening-gap-in-mortality-rate-between-the-u-s-and-peer-

3. Healthline. (2023, June 23). *What's the average weight for women?* Healthline.com. Retrieved September 23, 30 C.E., from

https://www.healthline.com/health/womens-health/average-weight-for-women

4. Motallebizadeh, N. (2023). Average Height in Japan 2023 - Limb lengthening center, Iran. *International Limb Lengthening Center of IRAN*. https://en.llcig.com/average-height-in-japan-2023

5. *BMC Public Health*. (2023, October 9). BioMed Central. https://bmcpublichealth.biomedcentral.com/articles/

6. Holland, K. (2019, June 12). *What is the average waist size for women?* Healthline. https://www.healthline.com/health/average-waist-size-for-women

7. Palavi Rao. (2023, July 13). *Mapped: Meat Consumption by By Country and Type.* https://www.visualcapitalist.com/. Retrieved September 30, 2023, from https://www.visualcapitalist.com/

8. Tanno, K., Yonekura, Y., Okuda, N., Kuribayashi, T., Yabe, E., Tsubota-Utsugi, M., Omama, S., Onoda, T., Ohsawa, M., Ogasawara, K., Tanaka, F., Asahi, K., Itabashi, R., Ito, S., Ishigaki, Y., Takahashi, F.,

Koshiyama, M., Sasaki, R., Fujimaki, D., . . .Okayama, A. (2021). Association between Milk Intake and Incident Stroke among Japanese Community Dwellers: The Iwate-KENCO Study. *Nutrients, 13*(11), 3781. https://doi.org/10.3390/nu13113781

9. Masayuki Otsuka, A. (2022, February 17). *Japan: Cheese Consumption Remains Stable Despite Pandemic Disruptions*. USDA Foreign Agricultural Service. Retrieved September 30, 2023, from https://www.fas.usda.gov/

10. *10 Popular Japanese Vegetables And The Unique Ways They're Used! | LIVE JAPAN travel guide*. (n.d.). LIVE JAPAN. https://livejapan.com/en/in-hokkaido/in-pref-hokkaido/in-sapporo_chitose/article-a0001413/

11. *Only 1 in 10 adults get enough fruits or vegetables*. (2021, February 16). Centers for Disease Control and Prevention. https://www.cdc.gov/nccdphp/dnpao/division-information/media-tools/adults-fruits-vegetables.html

12. Marion. (2017). What fruits and vegetables do Americans eat? More charts from USDA. *Food Politics by Marion Nestle.* https://www.foodpolitics.com/2017/05/what-fruits-and-vegetables-do-americans-eat-more-charts-from-usda/0/

13. Whittaker, R. (2023, July 23). World's biggest fruit eaters REVEALED in interactive map (and neither Britain or the U.S. is near the. . . *Mail Online.* https://www.dailymail.co.uk/health/article-12319805/Worlds-biggest-fruit-eaters-REVEALED-interactive-map-neither-Britain-near-bottom.html

14. *Japanese Fermented Foods | Lifestyle | Trends in Japan | Web Japan.* (n.d.). https://web-japan.org/trends/11_lifestyle/lif120223.html

15. *Japanese Fermented Foods: 6 great staples of a healthy diet.* (n.d.). Let's Experience Japan. https://gurunavi.com/en/japanfoodie/2016/12/japanese-fermented-foods.html?__ngt__=TT14a046ed3000ac1e4ae781vFVoQUPVjOCMVW6X8LLdsy

16. Taylor, B. C., Lejzerowicz, F., Poirel, M., Shaffer, J. P., Jiang, L., Aksenov, A. A., Litwin, N. S., Humphrey,

G., Martino, C., Miller-Montgomery, S., Dorrestein, P. C., Veiga, P., Song, S. J., McDonald, D., Derrien, M., & Knight, R. (2020). Consumption of Fermented Foods Is Associated with Systematic Differences in the Gut Microbiome and Metabolome. *MSystems*, 5(2). https://doi.org/10.1128/msystems.00901-19

17. Zava, T., & Zava, D. T. (2011). Assessment of Japanese iodine intake based on seaweed consumption in Japan: A literature-based analysis. *Thyroid Research*, 4(1), 14. https://doi.org/10.1186/1756-6614-4-14

18. Okumura, K. (2021, December 16). Please Don't Worry, Eating White Rice is Fine - Kaki Okumura - Medium. *Medium*. https://kokumura.medium.com/how-japanese-people-eat-so-much-white-rice-yet-stay-lean-4e1166d70f3c#:~:text=Japanese%20people%20eat%20lots%20of,lunches%20and%20in%20government%20cafeterias

19. Sakurai, M., Nakamura, K., Miura, K., Takamura, T., Yoshita, K., Nagasawa, S., Morikawa, Y., Ishizaki, M., Kido, T., Naruse, Y., Nakashima, M., Nogawa, K., Suwazono, Y., Sasaki, S., & Nakagawa, H. (2015).

Dietary carbohydrate intake, presence of obesity and the incident risk of type 2 diabetes in Japanese men. *Journal of Diabetes Investigation, 7*(3), 343–351. https://doi.org/10.1111/jdi.12433

20. *Nutrition - Health, United States*. (n.d.). https://www.cdc.gov/nchs/hus/topics/nutrition.htm

21. Tanaka, S., Yoneoka, D., Ishizuka, A., Adachi, M., Hayabuchi, H., Nishimura, T., Takemi, Y., Uneyama, H., Nakamura, H., Lwin, K. S., Shibuya, K., & Nomura, S. (2023). Modelling of salt intake reduction by incorporation of umami substances into Japanese foods: a cross-sectional study. *BMC Public Health, 23*(1). https://doi.org/10.1186/s12889-023-15322-6

22. Nutrition, C. F. F. S. a. A. (2022). Sodium in your diet. *U.S. Food And Drug Administration*. https://www.fda.gov/food/nutrition-education-resources-materials/sodium-your-diet#:~:text=Americans%20eat%20on%20average%20about,1%20teaspoon%20of%20table%20salt!

23. Koyama, T., Yoshita, K., Okuda, N., Saitoh, S., Sakata, K., Okayama, A., Nakagawa, H., Miyagawa,

N., Miura, K., Chan, Q., Elliott, P., Stamler, J., & Ueshima, H. (2017). Overall nutrient and total fat intake among Japanese people: The INTERLIPID Study Japan. *PubMed*, *26*(5), 837–848. https://doi.org/10.6133/apjcn.072016.11

24. *https://www.cdc.gov/nchs/data/nhanes/databriefs /calories.pdf*. (2000). Centers for Disease Control. Retrieved September 28, 2023, from

https://www.cdc.gov/nchs/data/nhanes/databriefs /calories.pdf

25. *Sugar consumption by country 2023*. (n.d.). https://worldpopulationreview.com/country-rankings/sugar-consumption-by-country

26. *Japanese Eating Habits | This month's feature | Trends in Japan | Web Japan*. (n.d.). https://web-japan.org/trends01/article/020403fea_r.html

27. Zulaikha, N., & Zulaikha, N. (2023). A Day of Ramadan 2023: Ramadan Experience of Muslims living in Japan | Food Diversity.today. *Food Diversity.today | Halal,Vegan&Vegetarian Information of Japan*. https://fooddiversity.today/en/article_134769.htm l

28. Baechle, J., MD. (n.d.). Intermittent fasting - the most popular diet in the United States. *www.linkedin.com*. https://www.linkedin.com/pulse/intermittent-fasting-most-popular-diet-united-jordan-baechle-md#:~:text=The%20IFIC%20showed%20that%20about,accounted%20for%209%25%20of%20diets.

29. Nomura, M., Yamaguchi, M., Inada, Y., & Nishi, N. (2023). Current dietary intake of the Japanese population in reference to the planetary health diet-preliminary assessment. *Frontiers in Nutrition, 10*. https://doi.org/10.3389/fnut.2023.1116105

30. Wright, J. (2003, April 17). *Intake of Calories and Selected Nutrients for the United States Population, 1999-2000*. Centers for Disease Control. Retrieved September 28, 2023, from https://www.cdc.gov/nchs/data/ad/ad334.pdf

31. Osler, T. (2023). Effortless Fitness: Why there are no gyms in Japan. *QOR360*. https://qor360.com/blog/effortless-fitness-why-there-are-no-gyms-in-japan/#:~:text=Japan%2C%20by%20contrast%2C%

20has%20about,'t%20like%20to%20exercise%E2%
80%9D

32. Bumgardner, W. (2022). What Is the Average
Number of Steps Per Day? *Verywell Fit*.
https://www.verywellfit.com/whats-typical-for-
average-daily-steps-3435736

33. Smith, L. (2023, January 6). *41 Exercise Statistics:
The Latest Fitness Trends (In 2023)*.
https://www.thegoodbody.com/. Retrieved
October 4, 2023, from
https://www.thegoodbody.com/fitness-statistics/

34. *10,000 steps a day: Too low? Too high?* (2020,
March 23). Mayo Clinic.
https://www.mayoclinic.org/healthy-
lifestyle/fitness/in-depth/10000-steps/art-
20317391

35. Rd, C. S. M. (2023, February 13). *9 Surprising
benefits of kimchi*. Healthline.
https://www.healthline.com/nutrition/benefits-of-
kimchi

36. Chisholm, A., MD. (2023, June 8). *How weight gain and weight loss affect your period*. Verywell Health. https://www.verywellhealth.com/changes-in-your-weight-and-missing-your-period-4105209

37. *Normal weight women: Avoid "Yo-Yo" dieting!* (2016, November 17). American Council on Science and Health. https://www.acsh.org/news/2016/11/17/normal-weight-women-avoid-yo-yo-dieting-10451

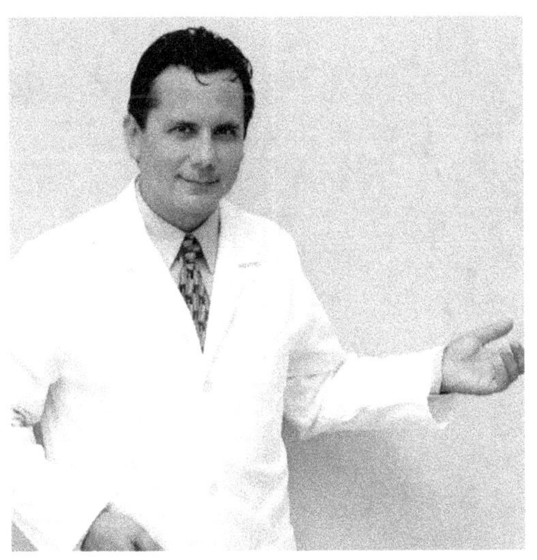

ABOUT THE AUTHOR

Rafael Bolio, MD, specialized in Internal Medicine, Critical Care Medicine, and Bariatrics. In 1990, while working in the National Health Program Fomento a la Salud, was instructed to create a viable nutritional strategy to be applied at the Mexican Institute of Social Security IMSS which provides medical attention to over 40 million people. He studied a population of over 10,000 office workers to identify the nutritional actions that were easiest to apply, and that favored better health. He worked with thousands of women going through menopause, which is when he discovered how his nutritional program practically eliminated menopause symptoms. The Secretary of Health later called for a debate with the country's experts in nutrition, and Dr. Bolio's plant-preferred nutritional approach was accepted as the most viable for the country.

www.ingramcontent.com/pod-product-compliance
Lightning Source LLC
Chambersburg PA
CBHW070840260726
48660CB00005B/2100